QuickFACTS™

Bone Metastasis

What You Need to Know—NOW

D1300758

*Quick*FACTS™

From the Experts at the American Cancer Society

Bone Metastasis

What You Need to Know—NOW

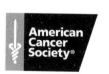

American Cancer Society®

Published by the American Cancer Society/Health Promotions
250 Williams Street NW, Atlanta, Georgia 30303 USA

Printed in the United States of America
Cover designed by Jill Dible, Atlanta, GA

5 4 3 2 1   08 09 10 11 12

Library of Congress Cataloging-in-Publication Data

Bone metastasis: what you need to know—now/from the
Experts at the American Cancer Society.
     p. cm.—(Quick facts)
     Includes bibliographical references and index.
     ISBN-13: 978-0-944235-81-2 (pbk.:alk. paper)
     ISBN-10: 0-944235-81-6 (pbk.:alk. paper)
     1. Bone metastasis—Popular works. I. American Cancer
Society.
RC280.B6.B675 2008
616.99′471—dc22

                                                    2007038361

A Note to the Reader

This information represents the views of the doctors and nurses
serving on the American Cancer Society's Cancer Information
Database Editorial Board. These views are based on their
interpretation of studies published in medical journals, as well
as their own professional experience.

The treatment information in this book is not official policy of
the Society and is not intended as medical advice to replace the
expertise and judgment of your cancer care team. It is intended
to help you and your family make informed decisions, together
with your doctor.

Your doctor may have reasons for suggesting a treatment plan
different from these general treatment options. Don't hesitate to
ask him or her questions about your treatment options.

For more information, contact your American Cancer Society
at **800-ACS-2345** or **http://www.cancer.org.**

Bulk purchases of this book are available at a discount.
For information, contact the American Cancer Society at
trade.sales@cancer.org.

Table of Contents

Treatment

Questions to Ask

After Treatment

Latest Research

Resources

Your Bone Metastasis

What Is Cancer?

Cancer* develops when cells in a part of the body begin to grow out of control. Although there are many kinds of cancer, they all start because of out-of-control growth of abnormal cells.

Normal body cells grow, divide, and die in an orderly fashion. During the early years of a person's life, normal cells divide more rapidly until the person becomes an adult. After that, cells in most parts of the body divide only to replace worn-out or dying cells and to repair injuries.

Because **cancer cells** continue to grow and divide, they are different from normal cells. Instead of dying, cancer cells outlive normal cells and continue to form new abnormal cells.

Cancer cells develop because of damage to **DNA.** This substance is in every cell and directs all its activities. Most of the time, when DNA becomes damaged the body is able to repair it. In cancer cells, the damaged DNA is not repaired.

*Terms in **bold type** are further explained in the Glossary, beginning on page 55.

People can inherit damaged DNA, which accounts for inherited cancers. Many times though, a person's DNA becomes damaged by exposure to something in the environment, like smoking.

Cancer usually forms as a **tumor.** Some cancers, like leukemia, do not form tumors. Instead, these cancer cells involve the blood and blood-forming organs and circulate through other tissues where they grow.

Often, cancer cells travel to other parts of the body, where they begin to grow and replace normal tissue. This process is called **metastasis.** Regardless of where a cancer may spread, however, it is always named for the place it began. For instance, breast cancer that spreads to the liver is still called breast cancer, not liver cancer.

Not all tumors are cancerous. **Benign** (noncancerous) **tumors** do not spread (**metastasize**) to other parts of the body and, with very rare exceptions, are not life threatening.

Different types of cancer can behave very differently. For example, lung cancer and breast cancer are very different diseases. They grow at different rates and respond to different treatments. That is why people with cancer need treatment that is aimed at their particular kind of cancer.

Cancer is the second leading cause of death in the United States. Cancer will develop in nearly half of all men and a little over one third of all women in the United States during their lifetimes. Today, millions of people are living with cancer or have had cancer. The risk of developing most types of cancer can be reduced by changes in a person's lifestyle, for example, by quitting smoking and eating a better diet. The sooner a cancer is found and treatment begins, the better are the chances for living for many years.

What Is Bone Metastasis?

Metastatic Cancer

Metastatic cancer is cancer that has spread from the part of the body where it started (called its **primary site**) to other parts of the body. When cells break away from a cancerous tumor, they can travel to other areas of the body through either the bloodstream or **lymphatic system.**

When the cells travel through lymphatic channels they can become trapped in **lymph nodes,** often those closest to the cancer's primary site. When the cells travel through the bloodstream they can go to any part of the body. Most of these cells die, but occasionally they don't. They settle in a new location, begin to grow, and form new tumors. The spread of a cancer to a new part of the body is called metastasis.

Even when cancer has spread to a new location, it is still named after the part of the body where it started. For example, if prostate cancer spreads to the bones, it is still called prostate cancer, and if breast cancer spreads to the lungs it is still breast cancer. A person with breast cancer that has spread to the bones is said to have breast cancer with bone **metastases.** (If you are talking about more than one metastasis, they are called metastases.)

When cancer comes back in a patient who appeared to be free of cancer (in **remission**) after treatment, it is called a **recurrence.** Cancer may recur in several ways:

- **local recurrence** (in or near the same organ in which it developed), for example, a recurrence of breast cancer in the skin of the chest near where the original cancer was removed;
- **regional recurrence** (in nearby lymph nodes or in the area from which lymph nodes had been removed); or
- **distant recurrence** (involving any other part of the body not included in local or regional recurrence). Distant recurrence is also called **metastatic recurrence.** For example, the cancer might recur in distant parts of the body such as in bones, the liver, or the lungs. This happens because some cancer cells have broken off from the original tumor, traveled elsewhere, and begun growing in these new places.

Sometimes metastatic tumors have already developed when the cancer is diagnosed. In some cases, the metastasis is discovered before the primary (original) tumor is found. Sometimes a cancer can spread widely throughout the body without developing as a large tumor in the site where it started. When the original site cannot be determined, this condition is called **cancer**

of unknown primary. To learn more about this condition, contact the American Cancer Society at **800-ACS-2345.**

Bone Metastasis: What It Means

Cancer cells that break off from a primary tumor and enter the bloodstream can reach nearly all tissues of the body. Bones are one of the most common sites for these circulating cells to settle and start growing. Metastases can occur in bones anywhere in the body, but they are mostly found in bones near the center of the body.

Bone metastasis is not the same as cancer that starts in the bone, which is called **primary bone cancer.** Bone metastasis and primary bone cancers are very different. Primary bone cancer is much less common than bone metastasis.

Information on primary bone tumors can be found in the American Cancer Society documents *Bone Cancer, Osteosarcoma, Multiple Myeloma,* and *Ewing Family of Tumors.* You can obtain these documents by calling **800-ACS-2345.**

Bone metastasis is one of the most frequent causes of pain in people with cancer. It can also cause bones to break and high calcium levels in the blood (calcium is released from damaged bones). Bone metastasis also causes other symptoms and complications that can lower your ability to maintain your usual activities and lifestyle.

Bone metastases develop in many people with cancer (except for those with skin cancers such as basal cell and squamous cell cancer) at some point in the course of the disease. The bone is the third most common site for metastases after lung and liver.

The spine is the part of the skeleton most commonly affected by bone metastasis. The next most common parts are the pelvis, hip, upper leg bones (femurs), and the skull.

What Are the Key Statistics About Bone Metastasis?

Of the estimated 559,650 people who will die of cancer in 2007, almost all will have metastasis. But certain cancers are more likely to spread to bone. These are breast, prostate, lung, kidney, and thyroid. In people with breast and prostate cancer, the bone is most often the first distant site where the cancer will spread. One expert estimated that about 350,000 people in the United States who die of cancer each year have bone metastases.

Risk Factors and Causes

What Are the Risk Factors for Bone Metastasis?

Risk Factors for Cancer

A **risk factor** is anything that increases your chance of getting a disease such as cancer. Different types of cancer have different risk factors. For example, unprotected exposure to strong sunlight is a risk factor for skin cancer, and smoking is a risk factor for lung, laryngeal, esophageal, oral, and several other types of cancer. Since a person must have cancer to have metastases, the risk factors for metastatic cancer are the same as those for cancer in general. These are the most significant lifestyle-related factors:

- tobacco use;
- an unhealthy diet;
- not getting enough physical activity;
- obesity; and
- alcohol abuse.

Together, the above factors are responsible for about two thirds of fatal cancers. **Genetic risk**

factors (inheriting certain **genes** that increase cancer risk) only account for 5% to 10% of cancers. About 6% of deaths from cancer result from exposure to cancer-causing substances in the workplace and pollutants in the environment. For more information on causes of cancer, please refer to information on specific types of cancer at the American Cancer Society Web site: **www.cancer.org**.

Risk Factors for Bone Metastasis

Bone metastases will develop in some people with cancer, but not in others. Doctors still don't know enough to predict for certain who will have bone metastases. But they do know that certain kinds of cancer are more likely to spread to bones. Among people with the same kind of cancer, tumors that are larger and have already spread to lymph nodes are generally more likely to have bone metastases. For some kinds of cancer, a high **grade** (the cancerous tissue appears very abnormal under a microscope) and certain genetic changes make the cells more likely to spread to bones.

Do We Know What Causes Bone Metastasis?

How Cancer Cells Spread

Metastasis is the end result of a multistep process in which cancer cells travel from the original organ in which they developed through the bloodstream and/or lymphatic vessels to reach other parts of the body. Understanding all the steps and learning how to prevent them is a major focus of cancer research.

Normal cells that make up organs such as the lungs and liver are held in place by a substance called **extracellular matrix** or **ECM.** This is not unlike the mortar holding bricks together to form walls of buildings. Except for blood cells, most normal cells in our body tend to remain in one place. The abnormal cells that form noncancerous (benign) tumors such as **fibroids** (leiomyomas) of the uterus, **adenomatous polyps** of the colon, and **fibroadenomas** of the breast are also held in place by ECM and usually do not spread to distant parts of the body.

Cancer cells are less dependent on their attachment to ECM. In most people with cancer, millions of cancer cells are probably shed into the circulation daily. However, just breaking loose is not enough. Cancer cells must be able to break through the walls of blood vessels or lymphatic vessels and then grow in their new environment. Most of the tumor cells entering the blood or lymphatic circulation are destroyed by the body's natural defense mechanisms or die on their own. Only those cancer cells that have become resistant to destruction and death will survive. Even then, the cells must be able to do several things normal cells don't do. Cancer cells must continue to be able to break through blood vessel and lymph vessel walls. They must then survive and grow in a new environment that is different from the organ in which the cancer developed. A key part of this growth is the cancer cells' ability to cause the body to build new blood vessels that will bring oxygen and nutrients to the cancer cells. This process is called **angiogenesis.**

Angiogenesis plays an important role in how cancer grows and spreads. A lot of research is being devoted to learning how to block this process with drugs.

Why Some Cancers Spread to Bone

Where a cancer metastasizes is influenced by its exact type and where it started in the body. Some cancer cells carry substances on their surfaces that cause them to stick to sites in different organs. Cancers that tend to spread to bone may attach better to the cells and supporting network (called **stroma**) in bone. In other cases, bone cells release hormone-like factors that cause cancer cells to grow faster. Recent discoveries about the interactions between cancer cells and normal bone cells are being used to develop new ways to treat or even prevent bone metastasis.

What Happens When Cancer Grows in Bones?

Often, the cancer cells make substances that damage the bones. Usually these substances can cause the bones to dissolve and weaken. This can lead to broken bones and large amounts of calcium being released into the blood, a condition called **hypercalcemia.** Sometimes, the cancer causes the bones to become harder, a condition called **sclerosis.** Both types of bone metastases can cause pain. When the cancer dissolves the bone, fractures often occur. Fractures occur much less often with cancers that cause sclerosis.

Prevention

Can Bone Metastasis Be Prevented?

For now, the only sure way to keep a cancer from spreading is to diagnose the tumor early enough and remove it with surgery or destroy it with radiation and/or drugs. The American Cancer Society recommends early detection tests for cancers of the breast, prostate, colon and rectum, and cervix. But some cancers may spread before they can be detected. There are many cancers that cannot reliably be found early by any of the tests we have now.

Researchers are studying ways to keep metastasis from occurring. For example, they are studying drugs that might block the **enzymes** that help cancer cells break through the walls of blood vessels. Recent studies indicate that a class of drugs known as **bisphosphonates** might slow the growth of bone metastases. These drugs are currently being studied to see if they can prevent bone metastases from developing.

Diagnosis

How Is Bone Metastasis Diagnosed?

The first symptom of bone metastasis is almost always pain. If you have cancer and begin to experience pain in a bone, you should report it to your doctor right away. Sometimes, if the cancer isn't promptly treated, the bone may break. Your doctor will want to x-ray the painful area and do **scans** or other **imaging tests.** Other diseases, such as bone infections and arthritis, or just being very active, can also make bones hurt.

When a cancer is first diagnosed, doctors will recommend a series of other tests to find out how far it has spread. Depending on certain features of the primary tumor (such as its size and exact type), your doctors will estimate your risk of metastasis and may recommend tests to search for it. If no metastases are found, then the primary cancer will be treated and you will see the doctor at regular intervals for follow-up care. One of the main purposes of follow-up care is to find out if the cancer is beginning to come back either at the original site or elsewhere at a metastatic site.

Symptoms of Bone Metastasis

The symptoms of bone metastasis can be mild at first. You may notice your appetite decreasing and

have trouble sleeping because you are uncomfortable. These symptoms can make it hard to
perform your usual activities.

Bone pain

Bone pain is usually the first symptom of
metastasis to the bone. The pain often comes and
goes at first. It tends to be worse at night and may
be relieved by movement. Later on, it becomes
constant and may be worse during activity. It is
important to tell your doctor about bone pain.
The bone might be so weakened that it will break.
This can often be prevented if the bone metastasis
is found early.

Fractures

Broken bones (fractures) can occur and cause
severe pain. They may keep you from moving
much at all. In some cases, a fracture is the first
sign of bone metastasis. The most common sites
of fractures are the long bones of the arms and
legs and the bones of the spine. Sudden pain
in the middle of the back, for example, is a
common sign of a cancerous bone breaking and
collapsing.

Spinal cord compression

Cancer in the backbone can press on the spinal
cord. The spinal cord contains nerves that allow
you to move and feel what happens to your body.
This is why pressure on the spinal cord is one of
the most serious complications of bone metastasis.
Not only can the pressure on the spinal cord
cause pain, it can damage your spinal cord so

that your legs become numb and even paralyzed. Sometimes the first symptom you may have of spinal cord pressure is trouble urinating because nerves from the spinal cord control the bladder.

Hypercalcemia

If the cancer has metastasized to many bones, you may develop hypercalcemia (high blood calcium levels caused by release of calcium from bones). This condition can cause nausea, loss of appetite, thirst, and extreme tiredness. If left untreated, hypercalcemia can even cause you to lapse into a coma.

For the reasons listed above, it is very important that you tell your doctors and nurses about any new bone symptoms or changes in old symptoms. Early detection and early treatment of bone metastasis can help reduce your chances of further problems later on.

Sometimes bone metastases are found before they have a chance to cause any symptoms. Signs of bone metastases may be found through laboratory and imaging tests (such as bone x-rays or **bone scans**) that are done when the doctor is learning the stage of your cancer (called **staging**), or in a routine checkup after treatment is finished.

Imaging Tests to Detect Bone Metastasis

X-rays

During staging or follow-up of a cancer, your doctor may get **x-rays** of your bones. These may show evidence of the cancer's spread to one or more bones. X-rays will not show bone metastases unless the cancer has destroyed about half of the bone's substance.

Bone metastases can change the appearance of bone in 2 ways. One way is when metastases dissolve some of the minerals in the bone, which makes the bone less dense. These are called **osteolytic** or **lytic metastases** and appear on x-rays as a dark hole in the gray-white bone image. Bones with osteolytic metastases tend to break very easily.

Other types of cancer, especially prostate cancers and some breast cancers, cause **osteoblastic** or **blastic metastases.** These make the bone appear denser (sclerosis). On x-rays, these metastases appear as spots that are whiter than the surrounding bone. This is the second way metastases can change the way bones look.

X-rays can also reveal fractures (breaks) in bones that are weakened by metastases.

Radionuclide bone scan

A **radionuclide bone scan** helps show whether a cancer has metastasized to bones. You will be given an injection of a radioactive substance called **technetium diphosphonate.** The injection itself is the only uncomfortable part of the entire scanning procedure. The amount of radioactivity used is low compared with the much higher doses used in radiation therapy, and this low level of radiation does not cause any side effects.

The radioactive substance is attracted to diseased bone cells throughout the entire skeleton. Areas of diseased bone will be seen on the bone scan image as dense gray to black areas called **hot spots.** These areas may suggest metastatic cancer. Arthritis, infection, or other bone diseases can also cause hot spots; however, the pattern of these diseases is usually different from the pattern caused by cancer. To tell the difference between these conditions, the **cancer care team** may use other imaging tests or perform bone biopsies. Bone scans can reveal metastases much earlier than regular x-rays. Not only are bone scans useful in spotting bone metastases, they can also track how metastases respond to treatments.

Sometimes bone scans fail to find areas of cancer spread to the bones. This happens most often if the metastases are osteolytic. In some patients, the scan may show no radioactivity in certain areas of bone that have already been destroyed by the cancer.

Computed tomography

The **computed tomography (CT)** scan is an x-ray procedure that produces detailed cross-sectional images of the body. Instead of taking one picture, like the usual x-ray, a CT scanner takes many pictures as it rotates around you. A computer then combines these pictures into an image of a slice of your body. The machine will take pictures of many slices of the part of your body that is being studied. This test can help tell whether your cancer has spread into your bones. It is especially important when the bone metastases are only osteolytic, since these metastases sometimes don't show up in bone scans. Often, after the first set of pictures is taken, you will receive an intravenous injection of a "dye" or radiocontrast agent that helps better outline structures in your body. A second set of pictures is then taken.

CT scans can also be used to precisely guide a **biopsy** needle into a suspected metastasis. For this procedure, called a **CT–guided needle biopsy,** you stay on the CT scanning table, while a radiologist advances a biopsy needle toward the suspicious area. CT scans are repeated until the doctors are confident that the needle is within the mass. A **fine needle biopsy** sample (tiny fragment of tissue) or a **core needle biopsy** sample (a thin cylinder of tissue about ½ inch long and less than ⅛ inch in diameter) is removed and examined under a microscope.

CT scans take longer than regular x-rays, and you need to lie still on a table for 15 to 30 minutes while the scans are being performed. But just like other computerized procedures, CT scanning is getting faster and your stay might be fairly short. However, you might feel a bit confined by the equipment in which you have to lie while the pictures are being taken.

The contrast dye will be injected through an **intravenous (IV) line.** A few people are allergic to the dye and get hives, a flushed feeling, or rarely, more serious reactions like trouble breathing and low blood pressure. Be sure to tell the doctor if you have ever reacted to any contrast material used for x-rays.

Magnetic resonance imaging

Magnetic resonance imaging (MRI) scans use radio waves and strong magnets instead of x-rays. The energy from the radio waves is absorbed and then released in a pattern formed by the type of tissue and by certain diseases. A computer translates the pattern of radio waves given off by the tissues into a very detailed image of parts of the body. Like a CT scanner, MRI produces cross-sectional slices of the body, but it can also produce images that are parallel with the length of the body. A contrast material might also be used in MRI scans, but less often than with CT scans.

MRI scans are particularly useful for looking at the spine and spinal cord. If your doctor thinks your cancer is pressing on your spinal cord, this is the best test to find out. MRI scans are a little more uncomfortable than CT scans. First, they take longer—often up to an hour. Also, you are placed inside a tunnel-like structure, which is somewhat confining. The machine also makes a mild thumping noise that bothers some people. Some testing centers will provide headphones with music to block out this sound. In general, most people tolerate the procedure well.

Positron emission tomography

Positron emission tomography (PET) is usually performed with glucose (a form of sugar) that contains a radioactive atom. A small amount of the radioactive material is injected into a vein. Cancer cells in the body absorb large amounts of this radioactive sugar. A special camera is used to detect the radioactivity. PET scanning is useful to see whether the cancer has spread to lymph nodes. PET scans are also useful when your doctor thinks the cancer has spread, but doesn't know where. PET scans can be used instead of several different x-rays because they scan your whole body. Newer devices combine a CT scan with a PET scan to better pinpoint the tumor.

Blood Tests to Detect Bone Metastasis

Serum tumor markers

Some types of cancer release certain substances called **tumor markers** into the bloodstream. Patients with these types of cancer may have blood tests at regular intervals to determine whether levels of these markers are rising. For example, high prostate-specific antigen (PSA) levels in a man who has already had surgery or radiation therapy for prostate cancer suggest the cancer may have come back or, especially if the levels are very high, may have spread to the bones. A high blood calcium level is another sign that the cancer may have spread to the bones.

Other blood tests

When cancer spreads to certain organs, it may damage the organ's cells or change the way they work. This process may produce certain substances that can be found by routine blood tests. For example, bone metastases often cause high levels of alkaline phosphatase. Although this substance is made by both the liver and bones, special chemical tests can be used to detect whether it comes from bone.

Urine Tests to Detect Bone Metastasis

Several substances are produced when bone is damaged. These are often secreted into the urine. One such substance that can be measured is called N-telopeptide.

Tissue and Cell Sampling Tests to Detect Bone Metastasis

If you have had cancer in the past, your doctor can usually diagnose metastatic cancer based on how the bone scan or other x-rays look. If any of your blood tests also suggest metastatic cancer, this makes the diagnosis even more certain. Because of this, biopsies are usually not needed. But if the diagnosis is not clear, your doctor will need a biopsy sample from the abnormal area to find out if it is cancer.

Needle biopsy

There are 2 types of needle biopsies: fine needle and core needle.

Fine needle biopsy or aspiration. With fine needle biopsy, a very thin needle and a syringe are used to take a small amount of fluid and small tissue fragments from the tumor. The doctor can aim the needle at a suspicious tumor or area that can be felt near the surface of the body. This type of biopsy of the bone is done only if the bone is weakened or if the cancer has spread into the soft tissue around the bone. The biopsy is done after numbing the area with a local anesthetic. It may be uncomfortable, but is not very painful.

There are times that the suspicious area cannot be felt or seen because it is deep inside the body. Or the suspected metastasis may be seen on an x-ray, but there is no lump that can be felt on the surface of the bone. In these cases, the needle can be guided by watching it during a CT scan.

Core needle biopsy. One approach your doctor might take is to do a standard **bone marrow biopsy.** In this procedure, the doctor puts a needle through the back of your pelvic bone after it has been numbed with local anesthetic. This can be moderately uncomfortable. A core of bone and marrow will be removed. Often, this test will show cancer even though cancer has not been seen on x-rays of the pelvis. The benefit of this approach is that it is simpler than trying to biopsy the suspicious sites because they may be hard to get at or cause pain. But if there is a real question about a particular area of bone, then it can be biopsied with a needle.

Usually, the doctor who performs a bone marrow biopsy uses x-rays or CT scans for guidance. The needles used for a core biopsy remove a small cylinder of tissue (about $1/16$ inch in diameter and $1/2$ inch long).

Surgical Bone Biopsy

Sometimes, needle biopsies don't provide an answer and a surgical biopsy is needed. In this procedure, called an **incisional biopsy,** the surgeon cuts into the bone to remove a small part of the tumor. This procedure is not done very often.

Treatment

How Is Bone Metastasis Treated?

Treatment options for people with bone metastases depend on where the primary cancer developed, to which bones it has spread, and whether any bones are severely weakened or broken. Other factors will also be considered, such as specific features of the cancer cells (in the case of breast cancer, for instance, whether they contain **estrogen receptors**), your general state of health, and which treatments you have already received.

Most doctors believe the most important treatment for bone metastases is treatment directed against the cancer. This is usually done with **systemic therapies.** Systemic therapies enter the bloodstream and can therefore reach cancer cells that have spread throughout the body. This is different from local therapies, which are directed at a single area. Systemic therapies include **chemotherapy** or hormone therapies, which are taken by mouth or injected.

Drugs called bisphosphonates (see section on bisphosphonates on pages 32–35) can help make diseased bones stronger and help prevent fractures. These drugs are used to supplement the chemotherapy or hormonal therapy for bone metastasis. If systemic therapy is successful, then the symptoms of the bone metastases will go away and new symptoms are not likely to develop soon.

Treating the bone problems may also be important. Local treatments such as radiation therapy can relieve the pain in a bone by destroying the cancer. Sometimes a bone such as your femur (thigh bone) might look as if it is close to breaking. To prevent this, your doctor will recommend surgery that involves placing a thin steel rod in the bone. It is much easier to prevent a damaged femur from breaking than to repair it after it has broken.

Systemic Therapy

This section begins with a summary of the types of systemic treatments used for patients with metastatic cancers. For more detailed information about treating metastatic cancer that has spread from a specific type of primary cancer, or for more information about advanced cancer, stage IV (4) cancer, or recurrent cancer, please call our toll-free number: **800-ACS-2345.**

Chemotherapy

Chemotherapy uses anticancer drugs that are usually injected into a vein or taken by mouth. These drugs enter the bloodstream and can reach cancer that has spread. Chemotherapy is used as the main treatment for some metastatic cancers such as lymphomas and germ cell tumors of the ovaries, testicles, or placenta. In many types of cancer, chemotherapy can be used to shrink tumors. This generally makes you feel better and reduces any pain you might have.

Chemotherapy drugs kill cancer cells but also damage some normal cells. Therefore, careful attention must be given to avoiding or reducing **side effects.** These depend on the type of drugs, the amount taken, and the length of treatment. Temporary side effects might include nausea and vomiting, loss of appetite, loss of hair, and mouth sores. Because chemotherapy can damage the blood-producing cells of your bone marrow, you may have low blood cell counts. Low blood cell counts can result in

- an increased chance of infection (caused by a shortage of white blood cells);
- increased bleeding or bruising after minor cuts or injuries (caused by a shortage of blood platelets); and
- **fatigue** (caused by low red blood cell counts).

Most side effects go away once treatment is stopped. There are remedies to prevent or control many of the temporary side effects of chemo-therapy. For example, an **antiemetic** is a drug that can prevent or reduce nausea and vomiting.

For more information on chemotherapy, please go to the American Cancer Society Web site, **www.cancer.org,** or call **800-ACS-2345** and ask for the brochure *Understanding Chemotherapy: A Guide for Patients and Families.*

Hormone therapy

Estrogen, a hormone produced by the ovaries, promotes growth of some types of breast cancer, particularly those types for which tests can detect estrogen receptors. Likewise, **androgens** such as **testosterone** (produced by the testicles) promote growth of most prostate cancers. One of the main ways to treat breast and prostate cancer is to block these hormones.

There are several types of hormone-blocking therapies. One strategy is to remove the organs that produce hormones. Removing the ovaries in women with breast cancer and removing the testicles in men with prostate cancer are **hormone therapy** options. Drugs are another option. Postmenopausal women can be given **aromatase inhibitors,** which block the small amount of estrogen they normally produce.

More often, drugs can be given to keep hormones from being produced. This is a common approach to hormone therapy for prostate cancer. Other drugs can be given to prevent the hormones from affecting the cancer cells. For example, drugs such as **tamoxifen** block estrogen's effects on breast cancers. Men can be given drugs such as **luteinizing hormone-releasing hormone (LHRH)**, which block testosterone production, and **antiandrogens**, which block the male hormone's effects on prostate cancer. Side effects depend on the type of hormone treatments used. Use of tamoxifen, for example, may result in hot flashes, blood clots, loss of sex drive, and increased risk of uterine cancer.

Immunotherapy

Immunotherapy is a systemic therapy that helps a patient's immune system recognize and destroy cancer cells more effectively. Several types of immunotherapy are used to treat patients with metastatic cancer, including **cytokines, monoclonal antibodies,** and **tumor vaccines.** Most of these are still experimental.

These treatments are discussed in detail in American Cancer Society documents on immunotherapy and the specific types of cancer for which this approach is useful. For more information on immunotherapy, please go to the American Cancer Society Web site, **www.cancer.org,** or call **800-ACS-2345** and ask for the brochure *Immunotherapy*.

Radiopharmaceuticals

Radiopharmaceuticals are a group of drugs that have radioactive elements. These drugs are injected into a vein and settle in areas of bone that contain cancer. The radiation they give off kills the cancer cells and relieves some of the pain caused by bone metastases. Some of the radiopharmaceuticals that are most often used are **strontium-89** (Metastron) and **samarium-153** (Quadramet). Other radiopharmaceuticals, such as rhenium-186, rhenium-188, and tin-17, are also being studied.

Radiopharmaceuticals are not used to treat early-stage, localized cancer (cancer that has not spread) or metastases to other organs of the body.

They are used only for cancer that has spread from another site to the bone.

If cancer has spread to many bones, use of radiopharmaceuticals is much better than trying to aim **external beam radiation** at each affected bone. In some cases, radiopharmaceuticals may be combined with external beam radiation aimed at the most painful bone metastases (see section on Radiation Therapy on page 29). Radiopharmaceuticals have the advantage over external beam radiation of being given in a single dose. This single treatment can reduce the pain for as long as 1 year. Retreatment is possible when the pain returns, although usually the pain is not reduced for as long as it was with the first treatment.

Radiopharmaceuticals work best when the metastases are osteoblastic. Osteoblastic means the cancer has stimulated the bone cells (**osteoblasts**) to form new areas of bone. These areas appear dense (white) on x-rays (as opposed to osteolytic lesions, which appear as dark areas or holes in the bones). Osteoblastic metastases occur most frequently in prostate cancer that has spread to bone. They are found less frequently in breast cancer that has spread to bone and even less frequently in most other cancers.

The major side effect of this treatment is a lowering of blood cell counts (white cells and platelets), which could place you at increased risk for infections or bleeding, especially if your counts are already low. Another possible side effect is a so-called **flare reaction,** in which the pain gets worse for a brief time before getting better.

Local Therapy

Radiation therapy

Radiation therapy uses high-energy rays or particles to destroy cancer cells or slow their rate of growth. Radiation therapy can be used to cure primary cancers that have not spread too far from their original site. When a cancer has metastasized to bones, radiation is used to relieve (palliate) symptoms. Radiation may prevent fractures once the bone has healed. If there is an impending risk of a bone fracture, radiation will not prevent it. Instead the bone must be stabilized with surgery (see page 31). If the bone is treated before it gets too weak, radiation therapy may help prevent later fractures.

The most common way to deliver radiation to a bone metastasis is to carefully focus a beam of radiation from a machine outside the body. This is known as **external beam radiation therapy.** To reduce the risk of side effects, doctors carefully determine the exact dose and aim the beam as accurately as they can to hit the target.

External beam radiation therapy

External beam radiation therapy for bone metastasis can be given as a large dose at one time, or in smaller amounts over 5 to 10 treatments. Most radiation oncologists (doctors who specialize in radiation therapy) prefer to give the radiation over several treatments. Both provide the same benefit in pain reduction but, when asked, most patients prefer the single-dose treatment. The advantage of the one-dose treatment is fewer trips for therapy and lower costs. The advantage of more treatments is that it reduces the number of patients who need retreatment (because the pain has come back) from about 18% to around 9%.

Each treatment for external beam radiation lasts only a few minutes. External beam radiation is an excellent option if you have 1 or 2 metastases that are causing symptoms. But if there are many metastases scattered throughout the body, treatment is more difficult. In rare cases, some patients can benefit from radiation therapy to either the entire upper or lower half of the body. A few weeks later, the other half of the body can be treated.

Although it is rarely used to treat bone metastases, another method of delivering radiation is to place (implant) metal rods or tiny pellets (sometimes called seeds) that contain radioactive materials in or near the cancer. This method is called **internal radiation, interstitial radiation,** or **brachytherapy.**

For more information on radiation therapy, please go to the American Cancer Society Web site, **www.cancer.org,** or call **800-ACS-2345** and ask for the brochure *Understanding Radiation Therapy: A Guide for Patients and Families.*

Radiofrequency ablation

Radiofrequency ablation involves use of a needle that carries electric current. The needle is placed into a particularly painful tumor that hasn't improved with radiation therapy. The electric current that destroys the tumor and relieves pain is delivered through the needle. This is usually done while the patient is under **anesthesia.**

Surgery

Although surgery to remove a primary bone tumor (one that started in the bone) is often done with the intent to cure, the purpose of surgically treating bone metastasis is to relieve symptoms. Bone metastases can weaken bones, leading to breaks that tend to heal very poorly. An operation using a metal rod or external device to stabilize the bone can prevent some fractures and, if the bone is already broken, can rapidly relieve pain and help the patient return to usual activities.

If you can't have surgery to reinforce a bone affected by metastasis (because of poor general state of health, other complications of the cancer, or side effects from other treatments), a cast may help stabilize leg bones to reduce pain and avoid the need to stay in bed.

Sometimes the cancer will spread to a bone in the spine. The cancer can grow enough to press against the spinal cord, causing **spinal cord compression.** If not treated immediately, this can lead to paralysis. Surgery can relieve the pressure on the spinal cord and prevent paralysis as well as help relieve the pain. Radiation therapy is another option. A recent study has found that surgery followed by radiation may be the best treatment.

Pain Medications for Bone Metastasis

There are effective and safe ways to treat pain caused by bone metastasis. In some cases, this may include treatments that kill the cancer cells (chemotherapy or radiation therapy), slow their growth (hormonal therapy), or reduce bone damage (bisphosphonates). If the treatment does not relieve your pain, you should not hesitate to ask for pain medicines.

You may not want to ask for or accept pain medicines such as opioids (morphine-like pain medicines) because you think you will become addicted or that the medicines will make you too sleepy to continue your usual activities. In reality, addiction rarely occurs, drowsiness can be controlled, and being free of pain can help you concentrate on the activities that are important to you.

If you are in pain and have been given prescription pain medicines, you should take them on a regular schedule. It works better to prevent the pain than to treat it once it starts.

For more information on management of pain, please go to the American Cancer Society Web site, **www.cancer.org,** or call **800-ACS-2345** and ask for the brochure *Pain Control: A Guide for People with Cancer and Their Families.*

Bisphosphonates

Bisphosphonates are a group of drugs routinely used to treat **osteoporosis**, a condition that weakens the bones. They have also proven useful in treating patients with cancer that has spread to the bones. Drugs in this category include alendronate, clodronate, etidronate, ibandronate, zoledronate, and pamidronate. Bisphosphonates are also used to treat patients with **multiple myeloma,** a form of cancer that starts in the bone marrow.

Bisphosphonates help reduce bone pain, slow down bone damage caused by the cancer, reduce high blood calcium levels (hypercalcemia), and lower the risk of broken bones. They are more effective when x-rays show the metastatic cancer is causing the bone to become thinner and weaker (osteolytic metastases). They are less effective in treating osteoblastic metastases (sclerosis).

Bisphosphonates may be taken by mouth or given through a vein. Because the digestive system does not absorb these drugs very well, and because they can cause irritation and ulcers in the esophagus, bisphosphonate treatment for bone metastasis usually is given intravenously, every 3 to 4 weeks.

The most commonly used drug is zoledronate (Zometa). However, ibandronate, which can also be given intravenously, may be as effective. Pamidronate is also commonly used used to treat bone metastases. Zoledronate has an advantage over pamidronate because it takes less time to inject. Studies have also suggested that zoledronate may reduce the risk of fracture somewhat better than pamidronate.

Clinical trials (or clinical studies) have reported the most common side effects of bisphosphonates to be fatigue, fever, nausea, vomiting, anemia (low red blood cell counts), and bone or joint pain. But the cancer itself or other drugs that the patients were taking may have caused many of these effects. Bisphosphonates may also cause arthritis-like joint pain and muscle pain. These can often be relieved or prevented with a mild pain reliever.

Recently, doctors have been reporting a very distressing side effect of damage to the jaw bones in patients receiving bisphosphonates. This side effect is called **osteonecrosis.** Patients complain of pain in the jaw, and examining doctors find that part of the bone of the upper or lower jaw has died. This can lead to loss of teeth in that area. Infections of the jaw bone may also develop. Doctors don't know why this happens or how to prevent it. So far, the only treatment has been to stop the bisphosphonate treatment and try to surgically remove the damaged bone. The only factor that doctors have found that increases the risk of this problem is having jaw surgery or having a tooth removed. Such procedures should be avoided while taking these drugs.

One way to avoid the above dental procedures is to maintain good oral hygiene by flossing, brushing, making sure that dentures fit properly, and having regular dental checkups. Any tooth or gum infections should be treated promptly. Dental fillings, root canal procedures, and tooth crowns do not seem to lead to osteonecrosis. Some oncologists recommend that patients have a dental checkup and have any tooth or jaw problems treated before they start taking bisphosphonates.

Clinical Trials

The purpose of clinical trials

Studies of promising new or experimental treatments in patients are known as clinical trials. A clinical trial is only done when there is some reason to believe that the treatment being studied may be valuable to the patient. Treatments used in clinical trials are often found to have real benefits. Researchers conduct studies of new treatments to answer the following questions:

- Is the treatment helpful?
- How does this new type of treatment work?
- Does it work better than other treatments already available?
- What side effects does the treatment cause?
- Are the side effects greater or less than the standard treatment?
- Do the benefits outweigh the side effects?
- In which patients is the treatment most likely to be helpful?

Types of clinical trials

There are 3 phases of clinical trials in which a treatment is studied before it is eligible for approval by the **U.S. Food and Drug Administration** (FDA).

Phase I clinical trials

The purpose of a phase I clinical trial or study is to find the best way to administer a new treatment and to determine how much of it can be given safely. The cancer care team watches patients carefully for any harmful side effects. The treatment has been well tested in laboratory and animal studies, but the side effects in patients are not completely known. Doctors conducting the clinical trial start by giving very low doses of the drug to the first patients and increasing the dose for later groups of patients until side effects appear. Although doctors are hoping to help patients, the main purpose of a phase I study is to test the safety of the drug.

Phase II clinical trials

Phase II studies are designed to see if the drug works. Patients are given the highest dose possible without causing severe side effects (determined from the phase I study) and then are closely observed to monitor the drug's effect on the cancer. The cancer care team also looks for side effects.

Phase III clinical trials

Phase III studies involve large numbers of patients—often several hundred. One group (the control group) receives the standard (most accepted) treatment. The other group receives the new treatment. All patients in phase III studies are closely watched. The study will be stopped if the side effects of the new treatment are too severe or if one group has had much better results than the other.

If you are in a clinical trial, you will have a team of experts taking care of you and monitoring your progress very carefully. The study is especially designed to pay close attention to you. However, there are some risks. No one involved in the study knows in advance whether the treatment will work or exactly what side effects will occur. The study is designed to find out this information. While most side effects disappear in time, some can be permanent or even life threatening. Keep in mind, though, that even standard treatments have side effects. Depending on many factors, you may decide to enroll in a clinical trial.

Deciding to enter a clinical trial

Enrollment in any clinical trial is completely up to you. Your doctors and nurses will explain the study to you in detail and will give you a form to read and sign, indicating your desire to take part. This process is known as giving your **informed consent.** Even after signing the form and after the clinical trial begins, you are free to leave the study at any time, for any reason. Taking part in the study does not prevent you from getting other medical care you may need.

To find out more about clinical trials, consult your cancer care team. These are some of the questions you should ask:

- Is there a clinical trial for which I would be eligible?
- What is the purpose of the study?

- What kinds of tests and treatments does the study involve?
- What does this treatment do? Has it been used before?
- Will I know which treatment I receive?
- What is likely to happen in my case with, or without, this new treatment?
- What are my other choices and their advantages and disadvantages?
- How could the study affect my daily life?
- What side effects can I expect from the study? Can the side effects be controlled?
- Will I have to be hospitalized? If so, how often and for how long?
- Will the study cost me anything? Will any of the treatments be free?
- If I am harmed as a result of the research, are there treatments to which I would be entitled?
- What type of long-term follow-up care is part of the study?
- Has the treatment been used to treat other types of cancer?

The American Cancer Society offers a clinical trials matching service for patients, their family, and friends. You can reach this service on our Web site at **http://clinicaltrials.cancer.org** or by calling **800-303-5691.** Based on the information you provide about your cancer type, stage, and previous treatments, this service can compile a list of clinical trials that match your medical needs. In finding a center most convenient for you, the service can also take into account where you live and whether you are willing to travel.

You can also get a list of current clinical trials by calling the National Cancer Institute's Cancer Information Service toll free at **800-4-CANCER** or by visiting the NCI clinical trials Web site at **www.cancer.gov/clinical_trials/**.

Complementary and Alternative Therapies

Complementary and alternative therapies are a diverse group of health care practices, systems, and products that are not part of usual medical treatment. They may include products such as vitamins, herbs, or dietary supplements, or procedures such as acupuncture, massage, and a host of other types of treatment. There is a great deal of interest today in complementary and alternative treatments for cancer. Many are now being studied to find out if they are truly helpful to people with cancer.

You may hear about different treatments from family, friends, and others, which may be offered as a way to treat your cancer or to help you feel better. Some of these treatments are harmless in certain situations, while others have been shown to cause harm. Most of them are of unproven benefit.

The American Cancer Society defines **complementary medicine** or methods as those that are used along with your regular medical care. If these treatments are carefully managed, they may add to your comfort and well-being.

Alternative medicines are defined as those that are used instead of your regular medical care. Some of them have been proven not to be useful or even to be harmful, but are still promoted as "cures." If you choose to use these alternatives, they may reduce your chance of fighting your cancer by delaying, replacing, or interfering with regular cancer treatment.

Before changing your treatment or adding any of these methods, discuss this openly with your doctor or nurse. Some methods can be safely used along with standard medical treatment. Others, however, can interfere with standard treatment or cause serious side effects. That is why it's important to talk with your doctor.

For more information about specific complementary and alternative therapies used for cancer, call the American Cancer Society (**800-ACS-2345**), or go to our Web site (**www.cancer.org**).

More Treatment Information

For more details on treatment options, including some that may not be addressed in this book, the National Comprehensive Cancer Network (NCCN) and the National Cancer Institute (NCI) are good sources of information.

The NCCN, which comprises experts from 21 of the nation's leading cancer centers, develops cancer treatment guidelines for doctors to use when treating patients. The NCCN does not have a specific guideline for bone metastasis. However, bone metastasis is discussed as part of several guidelines on various cancer types and in some of the **palliative treatment** guidelines. Those are available on the NCCN Web site (www.nccn.org).

The NCI provides treatment guidelines via its telephone information center (**800-4-CANCER**) and its Web site (**www.cancer.gov**). Detailed guidelines intended for use by cancer care professionals are also available through the Web site.

Questions to Ask

What Should You Ask Your Doctor About Bone Metastasis?

It is important to have open and honest communications with your doctor about your condition. Your doctor and the rest of your cancer care team want to answer all of your questions. Consider asking these questions:

- What treatment options do I have for relieving bone pain?
- What treatment choices do I have for treating or preventing broken bones?
- Which treatments do you recommend, and why?
- Is the treatment you recommend intended to cure the cancer, to help me live longer, or to relieve or prevent specific symptoms of the cancer?
- What side effects are likely to result from the treatment(s) that you recommend, and what can I do to help reduce these side effects?

After Treatment

What Happens After Treatment for Bone Metastasis?

Follow-up visits to the oncologist help judge how effective your treatments are and whether additional treatment will be useful. You should report any new symptoms to the doctor right away so that new metastases or side effects can be treated. Prompt diagnosis of any new metastasis may make treatment most effective. These follow-up examinations can also detect short-term and long-term side effects of treatment. Checkups usually include a medical history (interview concerning symptoms), careful physical examination, x-rays when necessary, and laboratory tests. Although doctors have general guidelines for follow-up of metastatic cancers starting in various organs, the exact schedule of examinations and tests depends on your specific medical situation.

Treatment can often help shrink bone metastases and relieve symptoms. But bone metastases are usually not curable. At some point for many people, treatment directed at the cancer may not be effective. There are other treatments that can relieve your symptoms and make you feel better. Talk with your doctor about your options for palliative care to be sure you get the best relief for the symptoms that bother you most.

For more information, call the American Cancer Society (**800-ACS-2345**), and ask for the brochure on *Advanced Cancer,* or go to our Web site (**www.cancer.org**).

Other Things to Consider

During and after treatment, you may be able to quicken your recovery and improve your quality of life by taking an active role. Learn about the benefits and disadvantages of each of your treatment options, and ask questions of your cancer care team if there is anything you do not understand. Learn about and look out for side effects of treatment. Report these promptly to your cancer care team so that they can take steps to minimize them and shorten their duration.

Remember that your body is as unique as your personality and your fingerprints. Although understanding your cancer's stage and learning about the effectiveness of your treatment options can help predict what health problems you may face, no one can say precisely how you will respond to cancer or its treatment.

You may have special strengths such as a history of excellent nutrition and physical activity, a strong family support system, or a deep faith, and these strengths may make a difference in how you respond to cancer. In fact, behavioral scientists have recently found that some people who took advantage of a social support system, such as a cancer support group, had a better quality of life. There are also experienced professionals in mental health, social work, and pastoral services who may help you cope with your illness.

If you are being treated for cancer, be aware of the battle that is going on in your body. Radiation therapy and chemotherapy add to the fatigue caused by the disease itself. Rest as much as you need to so that you will feel better as time goes on. Ask your cancer care team whether your cancer or its treatments might limit your exercise program or other activities. If not, find out what kind of exercise would be most helpful for you.

Cancer and its treatment are major life challenges, with effects on you and everyone who cares for you. Before you get to the point where you feel overwhelmed, consider attending a meeting of a local support group. There are many groups available that provide emotional support, friendship, and understanding. Your cancer care team can suggest other organizations that might help you during your recovery. If you need individual assistance or a referral to a mental health professional, contact your hospital's social service department or call us (**800-ACS-2345**) for help in contacting counselors or other services.

Latest Research

What's New in Bone Metastasis Research and Treatment?

As scientists learn more exactly how cancer cells break off from a main tumor, spread through the blood and lymphatic circulation, and begin to grow in a new location, they come closer to the goal of developing treatments that can prevent bone metastases.

Angiogenesis Research

Research in the area of angiogenesis (formation of blood vessels) is particularly exciting and may eventually lead to ways of preventing or treating metastatic cancer. Several drugs that can prevent the formation of new blood vessels that cancers need in order to grow and spread have been tested in clinical trials and found to be effective in certain cancers. More trials are in progress and new drugs are being developed.

Radiation Therapy

Use of radiopharmaceuticals is expanding, and researchers are studying new ways to specifically aim radioactive particles to cancer cells by combining them with antibodies or certain chemicals. The technology for accurate delivery of external beam and internal radiation therapy is constantly being improved.

Radiopharmaceuticals
Newer drugs are being developed that have fewer side effects such as bone marrow damage.

Targeted Therapies
We are learning how cancer cells are driven to grow by certain abnormal molecules inside the cancer cell. Many drugs are being developed to target these abnormal molecules and prevent their action on cancer cells. Several are close to being available for treatment. Likewise, we are learning that osteoclasts and osteoblasts contain specific molecules that can be targeted and affect bone growth.

New Tests
A special kind of PET scan for bone uses radioactive fluoride instead of glucose. The fluoride is attracted to bone metastases better than the glucose. It is especially useful with newer devices that combine a CT scan and a PET scan to even better pinpoint the tumor.

Search for New Drugs
Although they are not as close to being developed, a search for drugs that block the action of cancer cells on bone is underway. Cancer cells secrete chemicals that cause bones to dissolve. These chemicals are being identified, and it is hoped that drugs that block them will be developed.

Resources

Additional Resources

More Information from Your American Cancer Society

We have selected some related information that may also be helpful to you. These materials may be ordered through our toll-free number.

Advanced Cancer (also available in Spanish)

Advanced Illness: Financial Guidance for Cancer Survivors and Their Families

Helping Children When a Family Member Has Cancer: Dealing with a Parent's Terminal Illness

Helping Children When a Family Member Has Cancer: Dealing with Treatment

Home Care for the Person with Cancer: A Guide for Patients and Families (also available in Spanish)

Hospice Care

Nearing the End of Life

The following books are available from the American Cancer Society. Call us at 800-ACS-2345 to ask about costs or to place your order. See other books published by the American Cancer Society at the back of this book.

American Cancer Society's Guide to Pain Control

Caregiving: A Step-By-Step Resource for Caring for the Person with Cancer at Home

National Organizations and Web Sites

The following organizations can provide additional information and resources.*

National Cancer Institute
Telephone: 1-800-4-CANCER (1-800-422-6237)
TYY: 1-800-332-8615
Internet Address: www.cancer.gov

National Coalition for Cancer Survivorship
Telephone: 1-877-NCCS-YES (622-7937)
Internet Address: www.canceradvocacy.org

Inclusion on this list does not imply endorsement by the American Cancer Society.

The American Cancer Society is happy to address almost any cancer-related topic. If you have any more questions, please call us at **800-ACS-2345** at any time, 24 hours a day.

References

American Cancer Society. *Cancer Facts and Figures 2007*. Atlanta, GA: American Cancer Society; 2007.

Bamias A, Kastritis E, Bamia C. Osteonecrosis of the jaw in cancer after treatment with bisphosphonates: Incidence and risk factors. *J Clin Oncol.* 2005;23:8580–8587.

Coleman RE, Rubens RD. Bone metastasis. In: Abeloff MD, Armitage JO, Lichter AS, Niederhuber JE. Kastan MB, McKenna WG. *Clinical Oncology.* Philadelphia, PA: Elsevier; 2004:1091–1128.

Finlay IG, Mason MD, Shelley M. Radioisotopes for the palliation of metastatic bone cancer: a systematic review. *Lancet Oncol.* 2005;6:392–400.

Hartsell WF, Scot CB, Watkins D. Randomized trial of short- versus long-course radiotherapy for palliation of painful bone metastases. *J Natl Cancer Inst.* 2005;97:798–804.

Manoso MW, Healey JH. Metastastic cancer to the bone. In: DeVita VT, Hellman S, Rosenberg SA, eds. *Cancer: Principles and Practice of Oncology.* Philadelphia, PA: Lippincott Williams & Wilkins; 2005; 2368–2380.

Mundy G. Metastasis to bone: causes, consequences and therapeutic opportunities. *Nature Reviews Cancer.* 2002;2:584–593.

Pavlakis N, Schmidt R, Stockler M. Bisphosphonates for breast cancer. *Cochrane Database Syst Rev.* 2005 Jul 20;CD003474.

Glossary

adenomatous polyp (add-uh-NO-ma-tous PAHL-up): a benign growth starting in the glandular tissue. *See also* fibroadenoma.

alternative medicines (alternative therapy): an unproven medication or therapy that is recommended instead of standard (proven) therapy. Some alternative therapies have dangerous or even life-threatening side effects. With others, the main danger is that the patient may lose the opportunity to benefit from standard therapy. The American Cancer Society recommends that patients considering the use of any alternative or complementary therapy discuss this with their health care team. *See also* complementary medicines.

androgen (AN-dro-jen): any male sex hormone. The major androgen is testosterone.

anesthesia (an-es-THEE-zhuh): the loss of feeling or sensation as a result of drugs or gases. General anesthesia causes loss of consciousness ("puts you to sleep"). Local or regional anesthesia numbs only a certain area.

angiogenesis (an-jee-o-JEN-uh-sis): the formation of new blood vessels. Some cancer treatments work by blocking angiogenesis, thus preventing blood from reaching the tumor.

antiandrogen: a drug used to block the production or interfere with the action of male sex hormones.

antiemetic (an-tie-eh-MEH-tik): a drug that prevents or relieves nausea and vomiting, which are common side effects of chemotherapy.

aromatase inhibitors (uh-ROH-muh-tayz in-HIH-bih-ters): drugs used in the treatment of breast cancer in women who are past menopause. Aromatase inhibitors keep an enzyme called aromatase from converting other hormones into estrogen. Examples of aromatase inhibitors include anastrozole (Arimidex), letrozole (Femara), and exemestane (Aromasin).

benign tumor: an abnormal growth that is not cancer and does not spread to other areas of the body.

biopsy: the removal of a sample of tissue to see whether cancer cells are present. Biopsies are done in several ways. *See* core needle biopsy, fine needle biopsy, CT–guided needle biopsy, bone marrow biopsy, incisional biopsy.

bisphosphonates: drugs that are sometimes given to cancer patients whose disease has spread to the bones. When injected into a vein or taken by mouth, bisphosphonates can slow the breakdown of bone, lower the rate of bone fractures, and treat bone pain.

blastic metastases: *see* osteoblastic metastases.

bone marrow biopsy: a procedure in which a needle is placed into the cavity of a bone, usually the hip or breast bone, to remove a small amount of bone marrow for examination under a microscope.

bone scan: an imaging method that gives important information about the bones, including the location of cancer that may have spread to the bones. It can be done as an outpatient procedure and is painless, except for the needle stick when a low-dose radioactive substance is injected into a vein. Special pictures are taken to see where the radioactivity collects, pointing to an abnormality.

brachytherapy (brake-ee-THER-uh-pee): internal radiation treatment given by placing radioactive material directly into the tumor or close to it. Also called interstitial radiation therapy or seed implantation. *See* internal radiation. *Compare with* external beam radiation therapy.

cancer: cancer is not just one disease but a group of diseases. All forms of cancer cause cells in the body to change and grow out of control. Most types of cancer cells form a lump or mass called a tumor. The tumor can invade and destroy healthy tissue. Cells from the tumor can break away and travel to other parts of the body. There they can continue to grow. This spreading process is called metastasis. When cancer spreads, it is still named after the part of the body where it started. For example, if breast cancer spreads to the lungs, it is still breast cancer, not lung cancer. Some cancers, such as blood cancers, do not form a tumor. Not all tumors are cancer. A tumor that is not cancer is called benign. Benign tumors do not grow and spread the way cancer does. They are usually not a threat to life.

cancer care team: the group of health care professionals who work together to find, treat, and care for people with cancer. The cancer care team may include any or all of the following and others: primary care physicians, pathologists, oncology specialists (medical oncologist, radiation oncologist), surgeons (including surgical specialists such as thoracic surgeons and neurosurgeons), nurses, oncology nurse specialists, and oncology social workers. Whether the team is linked formally or informally, there is usually one person who takes the job of coordinating the team.

cancer cells: cells that divide and reproduce abnormally and have the potential to spread throughout the body and crowd out normal cells.

cancer of unknown primary: the diagnosis when metastatic cancer is found, but the place where the cancer began (the primary site) cannot be found.

chemotherapy (key-mo-THER-uh-pee): treatment with drugs to destroy cancer cells. Chemotherapy is often used, either alone or with surgery or radiation, to treat cancer that has spread or come back (recurred), or when there is a strong chance that it could recur. It is often called "chemo" for short.

clinical trial: a research study to test new drugs or other treatments to compare current, standard treatments with others that may be better. Before a new treatment is used on people, it is studied in the laboratory and often in animals. If these studies suggest the treatment will work, the next step is to test its value for patients. These human studies are called clinical trials.

complementary medicines: treatments used in addition to standard therapy. Some complementary medicines (and therapies) may help relieve certain symptoms of cancer, relieve side effects of standard cancer therapy, or improve a patient's sense of well-being. The American Cancer Society recommends that patients considering the use of any alternative or complementary therapy discuss this with their health care team, since many of these treatments are unproven and some can be harmful. *See also* alternative medicines.

computed tomography (computed tom-OG-ruh-fee): an imaging test in which many x-rays are taken from different angles of a part of the body. The images are combined by a computer to produce cross-sectional pictures of internal organs. This test is often referred to as a "CT" or "CAT" scan. *See also* CT–guided needle biopsy.

core needle biopsy: removal of fluid, cells, or tissue with a needle for examination under a microscope. A core needle biopsy uses a thicker needle than that used in fine needle aspirates to remove a cylindrical sample of tissue from a tumor. *See also* fine needle biopsy.

CT–guided needle biopsy: a procedure that uses special x-rays to locate a mass, while the radiologist advances a biopsy needle toward it. The images are repeated until the doctor is sure the needle is in the tumor or mass. A small sample of tissue is then taken from the mass to be examined under the microscope. *See also* biopsy.

CT scan or CAT scan: *see* computed tomography.

cytokine (SY-toh-kine): a product of cells of the immune system that may stimulate immunity and cause the regression of some cancers. Cytokines can also be produced in the laboratory and given to people to affect immune responses.

deoxyribonucleic acid (dee-ok-see-ri-bo-new-CLAY-ic acid): the genetic "blueprint" found in the nucleus of each cell. DNA holds genetic information on cell growth, division, and function.

distant recurrence: *see* recurrence.

DNA: *see* deoxyribonucleic acid.

ECM: *see* extracellular matrix.

enzyme: a protein that speeds up chemical reactions in the body.

estrogen (ES-truh-jin): a female sex hormone produced mainly by the ovaries, and in smaller amounts by the adrenal glands. In women, estrogen regulates the development of secondary sex characteristics, including breasts; regulates the monthly cycle of menstruation; and prepares the body for pregnancy. In breast cancer, estrogen may promote the growth of cancer cells.

estrogen receptors (ES-truh-jin rih-SEP-ters): proteins found in certain normal tissues as well as some cancer cells. The hormone estrogen binds to these receptors and may cause the cells to grow. The tissues affected by estrogen normally contain estrogen receptors; other organs and tissues in the body do not. Therefore, when estrogen circulates in the blood, it only affects cells that contain estrogen receptors.

external beam radiation: *see* external beam radiation therapy.

external beam radiation therapy: radiation that is focused from a source outside the body on the area affected by the cancer. It is much like getting a diagnostic x-ray, but for a longer time. *Compare with* brachytherapy, internal radiation.

extracellular matrix: the material outside cells that provides support and structure to tissue.

fatigue (fuh-TEEG): a common symptom during cancer treatment, a bone-weary exhaustion that doesn't get better with rest. For some, this can last for some time after treatment.

fibroadenoma: a benign tumor that is usually left untreated. A small tumor will often go away within several months, though larger ones may persist for a longer time.

fibroid (FY-broyd): a benign smooth-muscle tumor, usually in the uterus or intestinal tract. Also called leiomyoma.

fine needle biopsy: a procedure in which a thin needle is used to draw up (aspirate) samples for examination under a microscope. *See also* biopsy.

flare reaction: a sudden, temporary worsening of tumor-related symptoms following the start of treatment. Flare reaction does not mean that treatment is not working or that the cancer has progressed.

gene: a segment of DNA that contains information on hereditary traits such as hair color, eye color, and height, as well as susceptibility to certain diseases. *See also* DNA.

genetic risk factors: risk factors that are inherited from a parent. A risk factor is anything that may increase a person's chance of getting a disease such as cancer. Risk factors can be lifestyle-related or environmental, or genetic (inherited). Having a risk factor, or several risk factors, does not mean that a person will get the disease. Most cancers are not caused by genetic risk factors. If a patient has several family members with cancer, however, genetic testing may be considered. *See also* risk factor.

grade: the grade of a cancer reflects how abnormal it looks under the microscope. There are several grading systems for different types of cancers. Each grading system divides cancer into those with the greatest abnormality, the least abnormality, and those in between. Grading is done by a pathologist who examines the tissue from the biopsy. It is important because cancers with more abnormal-appearing cells tend to grow and spread more quickly and have a worse prognosis (outlook).

hormone therapy: treatment with hormones, with drugs that interfere with hormone production or hormone action, or the surgical removal of hormone-producing glands to kill cancer cells or slow their growth. *See also* tamoxifen, aromatase inhibitors.

hot spots: areas of diseased bone that show up on bone scans. The hot spots can be bone metastasis, but they may also be arthritis, infection, or other bone diseases.

hypercalcemia (hy-per-kal-SEE-mee-uh): a high calcium level in the blood, sometimes due to cancer cells causing the release of calcium from bones.

imaging test: a method used to produce pictures of internal body structures. Some imaging tests used to help diagnose or stage cancer are x-rays, computed tomography (CT) scans, magnetic resonance imaging (MRI), and ultrasound.

immune system: the complex system by which the body resists infection by germs such as bacteria or viruses and rejects transplanted tissues or organs. The immune system may also help the body fight some cancers.

immunotherapy (im-mune-no-THER-uh-pee): treatments that promote or support the body's immune system response to a disease such as cancer.

incisional biopsy: a surgical procedure in which tissue is removed and examined by a pathologist. The pathologist may study the tissue under a microscope or perform other tests. When an entire lump or suspicious area is removed, the procedure is called an excisional biopsy. When a sample of tissue or fluid is removed with a needle, the procedure is called a needle biopsy, core biopsy, or fine-needle biopsy (aspiration).

informed consent: a legal document that explains a course of treatment, the risks, benefits, and possible alternatives; the process by which patients agree to treatment.

internal radiation: treatment involving implantation of a radioactive substance; *see* brachytherapy. *Compare with* external beam radiation therapy.

interstitial radiation (in-ter-STIH-shul radiation): a type of treatment in which a radioactive implant is placed directly into the tissue.

intravenous (in-tra-VEEN-us) (IV) line: a method of supplying fluids and medications by using a needle or a thin tube (called a catheter), which is inserted into a vein.

local recurrence: *see* recurrence.

luteinizing hormone-releasing hormone (LHRH): a hormone produced by the hypothalamus, a tiny gland in the brain, that stimulates the production of sex hormones in men and women.

lymphatic system: the tissues and organs (including lymph nodes, spleen, thymus, and bone marrow) that produce and store lymphocytes (cells that fight infection) and the channels that carry the lymph fluid. The entire lymphatic system is an important part of the body's immune system. Invasive cancers sometimes penetrate the lymphatic vessels (channels) and spread (metastasize) to lymph nodes.

lymph nodes: small bean-shaped collections of immune system tissue found along lymphatic vessels. They remove waste, germs, and other harmful substances from lymph (a colorless fluid that bathes body tissues). They help fight infections and have a role in fighting cancer, though sometimes cancer spreads through them. *See also* lymphatic system.

lytic metastases: *see* osteolytic metastases.

magnetic resonance imaging (MRI): a method of taking pictures of the inside of the body. Instead of using x-rays, MRI uses a powerful magnet to send radio waves through the body. The images appear on a computer screen as well as on film. Like x-rays, the procedure is physically painless, but some people may feel confined inside the MRI machine.

metastases (meh-TAS-tuh-seez): plural of metastasis (*see* metastasis).

metastasis (meh-TAS-tuh-sis): cancer cells that have spread to one or more sites elsewhere in the body, often by way of the lymphatic system or bloodstream. Regional metastasis is cancer that has spread to the lymph nodes, tissues, or organs close to the primary site. Distant metastasis is cancer that has spread to organs or tissues that are farther away (such as when prostate cancer spreads to the bones, lungs, or liver). The plural of this word is metastases. *See also* primary site, lymph nodes, regional involvement.

metastasize (meh-TAS-tuh-size): the spread of cancer cells to one or more sites elsewhere in the body, often by way of the lymphatic system or bloodstream. *See also* metastasis, lymphatic system.

metastatic (met-uh-STAT-ick) cancer: a way to describe cancer that has spread from the primary site (where it started) to other structures or organs, nearby or far away (distant). *See also* primary site, metastasis.

metastatic (met-uh-STAT-ick) recurrence: *see* recurrence.

monoclonal (mah-noh-KLOH-nul) antibody: a type of protein made in the laboratory that can locate and bind to substances in the body and on the surface of cancer cells. Monoclonal antibodies are being used to treat some types of cancer and are being studied in the treatment of other types. They can be used alone or to carry drugs, toxins, or radioactive materials directly to a tumor.

MRI: *see* magnetic resonance imaging.

multiple myeloma: a type of cancer that begins in plasma cells (white blood cells that produce antibodies).

osteoblastic: causing the bone to become more dense.

osteoblastic lesion: an area of abnormal tissue in which the bone has become more dense. A lesion may be benign or malignant.

osteoblastic metastases: the spread of cancer cells to the bone, causing the bone to become more dense. *See* osteoblastic lesion.

osteoblasts: cells involved in the production of bone.

osteolytic (os-tee-oh-LIT-ik): causing the breakdown of bone.

osteolytic metastases: the spread of cancer cells to the bone, which causes the bone to break down.

osteonecrosis (os-tee-oh-nuh-KROH-sis): bone death and tissue damage, resulting from poor blood supply to the area.

osteoporosis: (os-tee-oh-puh-ROH-sis): thinning of bone tissue, resulting in less bone mass and weaker bones. Osteoporosis can cause pain, deformity (especially of the spine), and broken bones. This condition is common among postmenopausal women.

palliative treatment (PAL-e-uh-tive treatment): treatment that relieves symptoms, such as pain, but is not expected to cure the disease. Its main purpose is to improve the patient's quality of life. Sometimes chemotherapy and radiation are used in this way.

PET: *see* positron emission tomography.

positron emission tomography (PAHS-uh trahn ee-MISH-uhn tom-AGH-ruh-fee) (PET): a PET scan creates an image of the body after the injection of a very low dose of radioactive sugar (glucose). The scan computes the rate at which the tumor is using the sugar. In general, cancer cells use large amounts of the sugar. PET scans look at the whole body and are especially useful in taking images of the brain. They are becoming more widely used to find the spread of cancer of the breast, colon, rectum, ovary, or lung. PET scans may also be used to see how well the tumor is responding to treatment.

primary bone cancer: a type of cancer that starts in cells of the bone. Some types of primary bone cancer are osteosarcoma, Ewing's sarcoma, malignant fibrous histiocytoma, and chondrosarcoma. This is different from cancer that spreads to the bone from another part of the body (a different primary site).

primary site: the place where cancer begins. Primary cancer is usually named after the organ in which it starts. For example, cancer that starts in the breast is always called breast cancer even if it spreads (metastasizes) to other organs, such as bones or lungs.

radiation therapy: treatment with high-energy rays (such as x-rays) to kill or shrink cancer cells. The radiation may come from outside of the body (external radiation) or from radioactive materials placed directly in the tumor (brachytherapy or internal radiation). Radiation therapy may be used as the main treatment for a cancer, to reduce the size of a cancer before surgery, or to destroy any remaining cancer cells after surgery. In advanced cancer cases, it may also be used as palliative (noncurative) treatment. *See also* external beam radiation therapy, brachytherapy, palliative treatment.

radiofrequency ablation (RAY-dee-oh-free-kwin-see uh-BLAY-shun): treatment that uses electric current to destroy abnormal tissues. A thin, needle-like probe is guided into the tumor by ultrasound or CT scan. The probe releases a high-frequency current that heats and destroys cancer cells.

radionuclide bone scan (ray-dee-oh-NOO-klide bone scan): an imaging test that uses a small amount of radio-active contrast material given in the vein. The radioactive material settles in "hot spots," areas of bone to which the cancer may have spread, and shows up in the picture.

radiopharmaceutical (RAY-dee-oh-FAR-muh-SOO-tih-kul): a drug containing a radioactive substance that is used in the diagnosis or treatment of cancer and in managing pain from bone metastases. Also called a radioactive drug.

recurrence: the return of cancer after treatment. **Local recurrence** means that the cancer has come back at the same place as the original cancer. **Regional recurrence** means that the cancer has come back after treatment near the primary site. **Distant recurrence,** also called **metastatic**

recurrence, is when cancer metastasizes to distant organs or tissues after treatment. *See also* primary site, metastasis.

regional involvement or regional spread: the spread of cancer from its original site to nearby areas such as lymph nodes, but not to distant sites.

regional recurrence: *see* recurrence.

remission: complete or partial disappearance of the signs and symptoms of cancer in response to treatment; the period during which a disease is under control. A remission may not be a cure.

risk factor: anything that is linked to a person's chance of getting a disease such as cancer. Different cancers have different risk factors. For example, unprotected exposure to strong sunlight is a risk factor for skin cancer; smoking is a risk factor for lung, mouth, larynx, and other cancers. Some risk factors, such as smoking, can be controlled. Others, like a person's age, can't be changed.

samarium-153 (suh-MAYR-ee-um-153): a radioactive substance used in cancer therapy.

scan: a study using either x-rays or radioactive isotopes to produce images of internal body organs.

sclerosis (skluh-RO-sis): hardening of tissue. Also used to refer to osteoblastic (thickened) bone due to metastasis.

serum tumor marker: *see* tumor marker.

side effects: unwanted effects of treatment such as hair loss caused by chemotherapy, and fatigue caused by radiation therapy.

spinal cord compression: a condition that occurs when cancer cells grow in or near to the spine and press on the spinal cord and nerves. This results in swelling and reduced blood supply to the spinal cord and nerve roots. Spinal cord compression can cause some patients to lose bladder control or have trouble walking. If not treated right away, these limitations can become permanent.

staging: the process of finding out whether cancer has spread and how far, that is, to learn the stage of the cancer. The American Joint Committee on Cancer (AJCC)/TNM system is used for staging many types of cancer. The TNM system gives 3 key pieces of information:

- **T** refers to the size of the tumor

- **N** describes how far the cancer has spread to nearby lymph nodes

- **M** shows whether the cancer has spread (metastasized) to other organs of the body

Letters or numbers after the T, N, and M give more details about each of these factors. To make this information clearer, the TNM descriptions can be grouped together into a simpler set of stages, labeled with Roman numerals (usually from I to IV). In general, the lower the number, the less the cancer has spread. A higher number means a more serious cancer. The 2 types of staging are clinical staging, which is an estimate of the extent of cancer based on physical exam, biopsy results, and imaging tests; and pathologic staging, which is an estimate of the extent of cancer by direct study of the samples removed during surgery. *See also* grade.

stroma: the supporting tissue of an organ.

strontium-89 (Metastron): a radioactive compound that is absorbed by the bone. It is used to treat bone pain associated with prostate cancer.

systemic therapy (sis-TIM-ik therapy): treatment that reaches and affects cells throughout the body, such as chemotherapy.

tamoxifen (tuh-MOK-si-fin): (brand name Nolvadex) a drug used to treat breast cancer that has estrogen receptors (is estrogen receptor positive). After starting the drug, some women who have breast cancer with bone metastases may notice a temporary flare (increase in bone pain), which usually indicates the cancer is responding to treatment.

technetium diphosphonate: the radioactive substance that is usually injected into a patient's vein during a radionuclide bone scan. The radioactive material settles in "hot spots," areas of bone to which the cancer may have spread, and shows up in the picture. *See also* radionuclide bone scan, hot spots.

testosterone (tes-TOS-ter-own): the male hormone, made primarily in the testes. It stimulates blood flow, growth in certain tissues, and the secondary sexual characteristics. In men with prostate cancer, it can also encourage growth of the tumor.

tumor: an abnormal lump or mass of tissue. Tumors can be benign (noncancerous) or malignant (cancerous).

tumor marker(s): one of any number of different chemical substances in the blood and other body fluids used to detect and identify different cancers. Tumor markers are not very useful for cancer screening because other body tissues not related to a cancer can produce the substance. But tumor markers may be very useful in monitoring for response to treatment when a cancer is diagnosed or for a recurrence.

tumor vaccine: an experimental treatment for cancer, in which a patient's own cancer cells are injected into the blood of the patient, or mixed with the patient's white blood cells in the laboratory, and then returned to the patient.

U.S. Food and Drug Administration (FDA): an agency of the United States Department of Health and Human Services. The FDA is responsible for drugs, biological medical products, blood products, medical devices, and radiation-emitting devices, along with other products.

x-ray: one form of radiation that can be used at low levels to produce an image of the body on film or at high levels to destroy cancer cells.

Index

Books Published
by the American Cancer Society

Available everywhere books are sold and online at
www.cancer.org/bookstore

Information for People with Cancer

Site-Specific

ACS's Complete Guide to Colorectal Cancer

ACS's Complete Guide to Prostate Cancer

*Breast Cancer Clear & Simple: All Your Questions
   Answered*

QuickFACTS™ Colon Cancer

QuickFACTS™ Lung Cancer

QuickFACTS™ Prostate Cancer

Praise for *QuickFACTS™ Lung Cancer*:
"The ACS has achieved its goal of providing overviews
that tackle need-to-know issues and supply references for
additional follow-up information as desired.
Recommended." —*Library Journal*

Symptom Management

ACS Consumer Guide to Cancer Drugs, Second Edition

ACS's Guide to Pain Control, Revised Edition

Eating Well, Staying Well During and After Cancer

*Lymphedema: Understanding and Managing
   Lymphedema After Cancer Treatment*

Support for Families and Caregivers

Cancer in the Family: Helping Children Cope with a Parent's Illness

Caregiving: A Step-by-Step Resource for Caring for the Person with Cancer at Home, Revised Edition

Couples Confronting Cancer: Keeping Your Relationship Strong

Social Work in Oncology: Supporting Survivors, Families, and Caregivers

When the Focus Is on Care: Palliative Care and Cancer

Help for Children

Because . . . Someone I Love Has Cancer: Kids' Activity Book (5 twist-up crayons included)

Mom and the Polka-Dot Boo-Boo

Our Dad Is Getting Better

Our Mom Has Cancer (available in hardcover and paperback)

Our Mom Is Getting Better

Inspirational Survivor Stories

Angels & Monsters: A child's eye view of cancer

Crossing Divides: A Couple's Story of Cancer, Hope, and Hiking Montana's Continental Divide

I Can Survive (Illustrated)*

A "Mom's Choice Awards" Finalist! (2007)

Cancer Information

General

The Cancer Atlas (available in English, Spanish, French, Chinese)

Cancer: What Causes It, What Doesn't

Informed Decisions, Second Edition

The Tobacco Atlas, Second Edition (available in English, Spanish, French, Chinese)

Health Books for Children

Healthy Air: A Read-Along Coloring & Activity Book (25 per pack; Tobacco avoidance)

Healthy Bodies: A Read-Along Coloring & Activity Book (25 per pack; Physical activity)

Healthy Food: A Read-Along Coloring & Activity Book (25 per pack; Nutrition)

Healthy Me: A Read-Along Coloring & Activity Book

Kids' First Cookbook: Delicious-Nutritious Treats to Make Yourself!

Tools for the Health Conscious

ACS's Healthy Eating Cookbook, Third Edition

Celebrate! Healthy Entertaining for Any Occasion

Good for You! Reducing Your Risk of Developing Cancer

The Great American Eat-Right Cookbook

Kicking Butts: Quit Smoking and Take Charge of Your Health

National Health Education Standards: Achieving Excellence, Second Edition